THE BASIS OF BRAIN REHAB

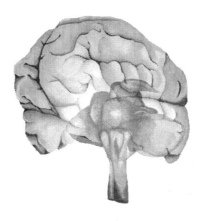

The author can be contacted at:

The Neuro Clinic:

1175 E. 3200 N.

Lehi, UT 84043

801-766-6580

office@theneuroclinic.org

ISBN: **978-1544070049**

Cover design: Matt Millette

Illustrations: Ryan Hatch

Chief Editor: Sarah Farmer

THE BASIS OF BRAIN REHAB

Acknowledgements:

I wish to give thanks to my sweet wife Becky who loves and supports me in all my endeavor's, to my chief editor Sarah Farmer, Christine Cook who challenged me to do this, and my belated mother who gave her life to helping special needs children and who pushed me to achieve educational excellence!

ABOUT THE AUTHOR

Dr. John D. Hatch is a successful business owner and the cofounder of The Neuro Clinic, a full service functional neurology center located in Lehi, Utah. Dr. Hatch is not only extensively trained but he is consistently inspired and creative in his approach to treating his patients. Dr. Hatch's tireless efforts to expand his work to benefit others has led to multiple patents pending. A rigorous work ethic, integrity, and a warm and friendly character inspire an immediate connection to Dr. Hatch from associates and patients. The nature of Dr. Hatch is to earnestly give his all to help others obtain optimal health.

Credentials:

Bachelor of Science in exercise science from Brigham Young University
Doctor of Chiropractic from Life Chiropractic College West
Diplomate of the American Chiropractic Neurology Board
Professional Applied Kinesiology
Fellowship in the American Board of Brain Injury and Rehabilitation

Dr. Hatch's family describe him as magnetic, joyful and energized. His closest friends know him to be honest, kind and compassionate. His colleagues appreciate him for being loyal, generous and devoted. His patients describe him as a passionate healer, remarkably intuitive and endlessly driven to serve and take on the most challenging cases. Dr. Hatch and his wife, Becky have two children.

CONTENTS

INTRODUCTION

Progress in medicine and science is
generating a greater understanding of the
connection between the body and the
brain. Advanced studies show that the
brain, gut, and emotions are interrelated
and affect many aspects of overall health.

Knowledge gleaned from these recent studies confirms that through functional neurology, improved brain function, overall health, and emotional well-being can be attained. The term functional neurology comes from "neurology," which is the study of the brain, and "functional," which means movement of a body part to create an action.

Functional neurologists study the brain's connections to the external world through sensory and motor systems and internal connections via reflexes, and the impact these have on the body as a whole.

Functional neurologists look for disconnects and dysfunctions in the brain and nervous system that cause a variety of health problems. Surgery and prescription medication is not part of the protocol. Functional neurologists repair the brain and body through exercises that stimulate targeted areas of the brain and central nervous system.

The Brain-Body Connection

Your brain is an incredibly complex organ that adapts to, reacts to, or causes everything experienced in life. Researchers seek to understand all of the brain's connections and its relation to the way people think, feel, act, and react.

Brain, gut, and emotional health are not often thought of as being connected.

- Stomach aches are often thought to be just a digestive problem.
- Emotional problems are considered a psychological issue.
- And with symptoms of movement or nerve disorders, such as hand tremors or seizures, doctors generally look for pathological brain lesions or tumors.

Pathological lesions are tissue or organ damage that can be seen on magnetic resonance imaging (MRI) or computed tomography (CT) scan images. Possible damage includes specific changes to brain tissue known as focal lesions, and/or degenerations (e.g., Alzheimer's disease or frontal lobe dementia).

In contrast, functional neurologists look for physiological lesions. Physiological lesions, a term coined by functional neurologists, describes *a neurological disconnect between one section of the brain to another.* A physiological lesion from the frontal lobe to the cerebellum, or from the motor strip of your brain that moves your hand, could cause a disconnect between the end organ and the nerves that activate the muscles that move the hand. These lesions are detected through a neurological examination.

Although all the above issues are often thought to be separate health conditions, functional neurologists look for ways they may be connected. For example:

- A constant stomach ache may be related to a visual problem, rather than just a digestive issue;
- Anxiety may be related to a gut issue or food allergy, rather than just being an emotional reaction; and

- A movement disorder may be related to emotions, rather than a brain lesion or tumor.

After locating physiological lesions in the brain, functional neurologists find ways to help the brain repair those disconnects—without surgery or prescription drugs, although those may also be needed.

Body Systems

The body has separate systems that work together in harmony to produce good health. The five governing bodies are: the nervous system, the enteric nervous system, the limbic system, the endocrine system, and the immune system. Here is a little more about them:

- The **nervous system** has two parts—central and peripheral. The central nervous system consists of the brain and spinal cord. The peripheral system is the nerves that branch out from the spinal cord or brainstem. The body has an estimated 37 trillion cells, all of which are trying to communicate through the body's nervous system.

- The **enteric nervous system** is made up of the gut and is highly connected to the nervous system. It regulates gastrointestinal function and has a mesh-like system of very intricate enzymes and molecule receptors.
- The **limbic system** comprises the hippocampus and amygdala, which are subdivisions of the brain. This system contains emotional experiences and memories.
- The **endocrine system** includes the pituitary, thyroid, adrenal, and reproductive organs. In other words, it is the hormone system.
- The **immune system** is located within the central nervous system. There are approximately 10 immune cells for every nerve cell, so most brain tissue is made up of immune cells.

The **vascular** and **lymphatic** systems are not included here, because they are not governing bodies. The vascular system is the messenger and carrier of information.

The lymphatic system helps the body eliminate waste and toxins. These two systems are regulated and controlled by at least one of the five governing systems.

Traditional medicine tends to separate all of these systems. However, the central nervous system is the check and balance system of the body—much like the judicial system. It is always balancing and checking what the immune, enteric, limbic, and endocrine systems are doing. This is the big picture to remember—*the central nervous system regulates all the other systems*. So, the question is, what really needs to be healed and what do people need to focus on to have optimal health?

Central Balance

This booklet outlines the reasons why people need to focus on rehabbing their central nervous system to obtain optimal health. Once that function is restored or developed, the brain enables the gut, hormones, immune system, coordination, and blood flow to function at peak levels.

This balance of systems then allows people to not only experience life, but to *enjoy it*. It also helps stabilize emotional well-being so people don't suffer from depression, anxiety, or other challenging emotional disorders.

The purpose of this booklet is to explain how the central nervous system works and, as the key governing system, helps people achieve their best possible health.

NEURON THEORY

The Role of Neurons

A neuron is a single cell that communicates from one cell to the next. The brain contains more than one billion neurons, and the body has multiple types of cells. When a neuron cell is activated by a nerve impulse (an electrical signal), it might activate a single other neuron, two neurons, or even

10 or 15 neurons. You may be asking, "Why is this important?" It is critical to understand, because when one neuron cell is activated, it doesn't just connect to another one in a direct, linear fashion. Instead, when one neuron is activated, it in turn activates multiple neuron pools around itself. Once one neuron cell is activated, it can activate 10, 15, or 20 other areas—meaning it spreads. Then those areas can activate another 10 to 15 areas, and so on and so on. This means *it is possible to connect parts of the body that have not been communicating.*

For instance, a person who has a brain area that isn't working due to a stroke can regain brain function. Although there may be an area that can't be activated due to brain damage, the areas around it can be. Then, in time, projections (i.e., expansion of activated neurons) can begin to reactivate the brain area that has been damaged, and changes can occur in that area. One way to think about this process is to compare it to a highway. We know the fastest route to a destination is a freeway. But if the freeway has traffic or road work, there are alternate routes to get to your destination. Those routes, over time, can become faster than the original freeway, or a new highway may even be built.

As an example of how normal pathways in the body can have scattered projections, think of the way your whole body jumps when you touch your finger on something with static charge, or the way your body shakes when you get the chills. These reactions happen because you have activated one sensory projection, which then connects to a bunch of other neuron pools. Those pools are connected to other sensory and motor systems, which create reactions to more than that one sensory stimuli. In most instance, when you touch something with your finger, the sensory nerve will connect to one neuronal pool up to the brain and create a single reaction or reflex. But when there is damage, or things aren't working properly, the sensory input will connect to multiple sensory systems and create other bodily reactions, such as if you ask a person to tap her fingers, and she also moves her arms, feet, or mouth.

Most neurons are activated by the body's external senses. As noted before, the central nervous system communicates heavily within itself. The peripheral nervous system sends all the information and feedback from your external environment into your central nervous system. The central nervous system's job is then to manage all the other systems. The sensory nerve cells of the peripheral nervous system are what tell the central nervous system what you are doing and feeling. For instance, are you spinning? Moving? Hungry? Angry? Sick? After receiving sensory input, the central nervous system interprets those inputs, regulates and checks with other sensory information, and then causes the brain to act or react. However, due to imbalances from the sensory system or central nervous system, these brain actions sometimes produce changes to your health.

When you are first born, certain cell types are already programmed and developed. Some cell types (alpha) receive sensory input, and some cell types (beta) receive motor input. Most sensory input goes back to the brain through a peripheral neuron that tells the brain what is happening. A message the brain might receive is, "My toe is getting pinched." The brain then sends a motor neuron down to the foot to move the toe. Some motor neurons are activated at the spinal cord level, such as a reflex, and not directly from the brain's motor system. An example of this is when you touch a hot pan and immediately pull your hand away due to heat and pain. Other messages must travel all the way up to the brain and then back down.

Peripheral Nerves

All the peripheral nerves go through the hands, arms, feet, legs, and body and feed information into the spinal cord. That information then travels up to the cerebellum (a subdivision of the brain), which provides balance and coordination.

This information then travels up to the final destination, which is the cortex, where you interpret and make sense of everything you experience. The cortex then sends a second relay of information to the cerebellum before making a decision of action; this process is done because the cerebellum is the mathematical genius of the brain. The cerebellum must know how all movements connect with each other. For example, when you tilt you head to one side and then point somewhere with your finger, your cerebellum must coordinate the weight of your head, the roll of your eyes, the neck muscles, the spinal muscles, and even your toe muscles, to keep you balanced and upright.

However, the peripheral nerves aren't just from the neck down. There are 12 peripheral cranial nerves that give direct input into the brain stem and then link to the cerebellum. Cranial nerves involving the eyes and vestibular apparatus (which detects rotational or linear movement) highly impact your balance. They provide the awareness of where your head and body are in space. These cranial nerves are crucial to regulating heart rate, blood pressure, oxygen, gut motility, digestive enzymes, saliva glands, moisture for the eyes, smells, and senses.

The most vital information shared between the peripheral nervous system and the central nervous system relates to gravity. The constant gravitational pull on your body enables your muscles to hold your body upright. The gravitational pull also activates the central nervous system and keeps it alive. For example, you get input from your feet when standing, and the muscles of the entire skeletal system sends information back to the brain via the nerves. That's why most people don't sleep standing up. When we lie down, we receive less muscle input to the brain via the cerebellum, which allows us to relax and then sleep. Lying down doesn't stop gravity working against the muscles, it just leads to less input from the major muscles and more input from the jaw and from when you shift or roll during the night. This way your brain and brainstem still receive enough information to keep you sleeping, breathing, and repairing. All body tissue grows and repairs best and fastest while you are sleeping, because growth hormones is released and the tissues don't have to deal with stimuli and the functions required of them.

The Role of Stimulation

Stimulation is constant in our lives. Most people get a lot of visual stimulation, but not as much movement. Every day, gravity works to provide stimulation to the body and give information to the central nervous system through the peripheral system. Have you wondered why people have chronic shoulder soreness, or ankle discomfort, or back pain, or headaches? The reason is because the peripheral system is giving the feedback to the central nervous system, but it isn't adapting to it properly or isn't receiving the signal in the right way.

Central neuron theory shows that every single neuron activates or excites (i.e., one neuron excites another neuron, and so on). Once a neuron is brought to threshold (meaning the action potential, which is an electrical gradient system that makes a cell excite), it hits a point that causes the nerves to fire. Simply put, once a neuron excites enough to fire, it sends a direct signal to another area. Once areas are stimulated, they either inhibit (stop something from occurring) or excite (cause the action to happen). This means you could *excite* a neuron that actually *inhibits* movement. For instance, when you touch your finger to your nose, your brain must excite the bicep to move while also inhibiting the triceps so the elbow can bend. The brain must then stop the bicep from contracting so you don't poke your nose too hard or punch yourself in the face; the brain does this by activating the triceps, which inhibit the bicep. For this movement to be smooth and coordinated, you need to know exactly where your finger, elbow, and shoulder are in relation to your nose. This one example shows how complicated movement is, and how many calibrations or calculations are needed to perform just one motion. The best part is that the brain does all this subconsciously and makes corrections without you giving it much thought.

Regulating Stimulation: Activation and Inhibition

Inhibitory nerve action is a great concept, because people often think they need to shut down input to achieve a desired outcome. However, you can often actually stimulate something in order to inhibit an area that has too much stimulation. For example, with headaches it is often thought that light and sound must be removed to dampen sensory input to certain areas of the brain. This can help get rid of the headache, but other areas of the peripheral system can be excited to activate an inhibitory neuron that helps alleviate the headache. For example, rubbing the forehead and neck is a common practice that can help get rid of a headache because of the touch or muscle activation these nerve connections make to the brainstem.

Neurotransmitters are what help cells communicate with each other, and most inhibitory neurons are *regulated* by a neurotransmitter called gaba. Gaba is primarily made in the cerebellum, the part of the brain that receives all input from movement. This means that as the body moves, there are increases in cerebellum activation, gaba production, and inhibitory neurons. The primary neurotransmitter used to *activate* communication from one cell to another is acetyl-choline. All other neurotransmitters, such as glutamate, serotonin, histamine, and dopamine, are excitatory neurons. Although histamine is excitatory, it is a proinflammatory neuron; this is why it can create chronic inflammation.

To keep your system balanced both with activation and inhibition, movement is needed. Movement is life. If you continue to move your body, it helps your brain function better. This is because the movement leads to more brain activation via the cerebellum, which then increases the inhibitory neurotransmitter gaba, which helps decrease overstimulation. But what about those who are in such chronic pain that movement hurts? That pain makes the idea of increasing movement hard to embrace. Thus, every practitioner who is working to improve a person's health needs to look at how to decrease inflammation and change the chronic pain response.

The Role of Nutrition

When looking at neuron theory, it is vital to think about the original cell. Every cell needs three things—oxygen, fuel, and stimulation. As long as people are alive, they breathe. Therefore, oxygen stays constant. Fuel comes from food that is eventually digested and broken down into simple glucose, protein (which is further broken down into amino acid), or fat. Another necessary fuel is water. It is very important to stay hydrated with good old-fashioned water (not soda).

Although nutrition is not the focus of this booklet, food is a very important aspect of body and brain health, as stimulation comes from all our senses. To learn more about eating properly for brain health, see the list of suggested reading at the end of this booklet. The big-picture recommendation is to eliminate processed or pro-inflammatory foods (e.g., genetically modified organisms [GMOs], artificial flavoring, dairy, corn). But don't just remove unhealthy foods from your diet; fill your gut with rich or dense nutrient-based foods, such as lean proteins, legumes, fruits, and vegetables.

22   THE BASIS OF BRAIN REHAB

HOMEOSTASIS

What is homeostasis?

Homeostasis is the body's ability to balance itself and its many functions. It is what allows the body to control its temperature, maintain the right balance of water and salt, and regulate blood pressure, blood sugar, and heart rate. As an example, the kidneys use homeostasis to balance the amount of water a person drinks with the amount that is released through urine. If the body has too much water, the kidneys put out more urine to balance the body out. And if a person is dehydrated, the kidneys conserve water and produce less urine. Homeostasis also helps cells balance the amount of salt and water they bring in, based on the ratio they need. This is important, because if cells don't have enough salt, they can't retain the water needed to function and circulate fluids. But too much water disrupts cell function and makes the body retain salt. Thus, balancing sodium and water levels is a function of homeostasis that keeps cells and the body healthy and functioning the right way. But there is much more to cell stability than just water and salt. Potassium, magnesium, and calcium also play key roles in a cell's health and balanced state.

How do homeostasis and chronic pain relate?

It is important to know that balance and health don't always mean the same thing, especially in the human body. The body and brain can be balanced or stable, yet not produce the desired outcomes of health. As one example, homeostasis plays a huge role for those in chronic pain. The brain is always trying to balance and regulate itself. For example, at this very moment, you are receiving pain signals from your peripheral nerves. All humans have pain cells and muscle fiber cells that send feedback to the brain. When you sit on a muscle, it has a pain cell that sends a message to the brain, but that signal is very slow. Because the action of the muscle signal is usually faster, it blocks the pain signal in the brain. This is called the pain gate theory.

Pain is only perceived in the brain, not the rest of the body, so if the pain signal does not reach certain portions of the central nervous system in the brain, the pain is not perceived. Yet if pain gate theory is true, why do some people feel chronic pain, especially when they move, such as those with fibromyalgia? There are many possible reasons for this. One reason may be a lack of serotonin that serves to block pain. This lack can occur when a brain is emotionally wound up, such as in people with post-traumatic stress disorder (PTSD). Another reason can be a lack of vitamin E that promotes healthy brain tissue. It may also simply be because the parietal primary sensory cortex (the sensory map of the body) in the brain has been distorted and needs retraining.

There are six different locations in the cortex where pain is perceived. Three of these are emotional centers in the limbic system. This is why physical pain is often associated with emotions, and why visiting with a therapist or psychiatrist can reduce chronic pain, such as in the neck, shoulder, or back, without the body ever being touched.

Another reason people feel chronic pain is because the brain has a hierarchy, meaning it perceives that certain body functions and responses are more important than others. Thus, it places first priority on the functions that ensure survival. This hierarchy is a hard concept to grasp. No one wants to feel pain, but the subconscious brain (or involuntary nervous system) does as it chooses. It is a common theory that humans can only use or tap into 10 percent of the brain. This theory is both correct and absolutely incorrect. Humans can only consciously control 10 percent of the brain, and the other 90 percent is involuntary, meaning you don't have control over it. This means some behavioral traits are an involuntary result or act, not a choice, such as tics, physical and emotional outbursts, emotional withdraws, and tremors.

The important thing to know is that this 90 percent of the brain is working constantly. You should be extremely grateful for this auto-pilot system, because if it was up to the conscious mind to heal a wound, breathe correctly, or breakdown food properly, most of us would likely die within 24 hours. But because of the brain's hierarchy of needs, the subconscious brain is more focused on balancing other systems of the body than on blocking chronic pain. Reducing pain is not a priority of survival, which is why most people can push through different levels of pain without stopping what they are doing. Also, the subconscious brain is continually making connections within itself, trying to adjust to constant change. For those in chronic pain, more of those connections are wound to pain neurons, so to get rid of chronic pain, the brain needs to be altered.

Brain Hierarchy

To look at homeostasis and chronic pain in greater depth, a few questions must be asked about the hierarchy of the brain. First, what is the most important thing for the brain? Given that death results when a brain goes without oxygen for an extended period of time, oxygen is the most important input to the brain. In fact, most people die if oxygen is deprived for just 5 minutes. Second, what role does gravity play? Astronauts who go into outer space don't get the necessary stimulation from gravity. Without this stimulation, their muscles and bones atrophy quickly. Space exploration has shown that gravity gives information to muscles and bones about how strong they must be. Thus, gravity is important. Another question to ask is,

"What about fuel?" Humans can fast and go without food for 1 or even 2 weeks, but without water, the average person will not survive very long—no longer than 3 days. Therefore, oxygen, gravity, and water are all necessary for proper brain function and human survival, so the brain places a higher priority on survival than on comfort.

In relating this hierarchy to homeostasis, the brain determines it is okay to have pain in the shoulder as long as there is enough feedback to balance the body's heart rate, oxygen, and vascular system, which are all involved with the fuel needed for every cell. Most people's survival system works well, so their brain can focus on balancing pain signals—this is why most people don't have chronic pain. Think of it this way: if the shoulder must shift to a position of pain to be more stable and keep the body balanced, then the brain chooses pain over instability. This change in shoulder position will then cause the vascular system to push blood to one area more than another, which affects fuel delivery to the lesser blood flow portion and may increase pain.

Headaches are a great example of this vascular imbalance that can be caused from multiple areas. Neck or head trauma can pinch or damage arteries to the brain, causing change in blood flow from one side to another. Even tight or stiff neck muscles on one side will increase more blood flow to those muscles and less to the other side or to the antagonist muscles. Over time, the lack of blood flow and fuel can promote tissue damage, because tissues don't have the fuel needed for repair. In short, fuel delivery is more important than blocking pain, which is why brain hierarchy is a very important concept when talking about chronic pain.

Sometimes the brain gets in a wound-up state in which it is so excited or overly active that it starts to cause tissue damage in other places, leading to chronic pain or trigger-point pain that never seems to go away. The reason the pain doesn't stop is because it's constantly being stimulated. A wound-up brain can also be related to emotional imbalances and learning disabilities. But again, this is the brain creating hierarchy.

Think of the chronic tender, tight, and often painful trigger points in your shoulders, or between your shoulder blades or neck. Those muscles are both phasic (voluntary) and postural (involuntary), meaning you can lift your shoulders or tilt your head left and right using your upper trapezius muscle, but you can't tell the little muscles of the neck to contract to make your head tilt—this motion is done involuntarily. You don't want the pain there, so why is it constant? The pain is there because the neck muscles that attach all these bones together (i.e., the skull to shoulders, neck to shoulders, and neck to skull) are activating via two major reflexes that are connected to the eyes and the inner ear, which sense movement. If the head is turned to the left, it causes the neck muscles on that side to constantly activate, and those on the other side to not activate. Over time this causes muscles in the neck to hypertrophy (get bigger) on one side and atrophy (smaller or diminish) on the other, giving more input from the activated muscles and causing the brain wind-up to continue. Hence the phrase chronic, or lasting, pain. In this instance, to repair the damage, the two governing reflexes in the ears and eyes must be fixed.

A simple example to illustrate this point is when you use your right hand to ring a doorbell. At that moment, your left cortex communicates with your right cerebellum to coordinate the movement. But the left cortex must send signals down the left-side brain stem, which then coordinates the posture of the left side to prevent you from falling over. This means that if you have difficulty pressing the doorbell button, you may have a problem in any one of those systems and the many subdivisions of the brain.

In summary, the brain is constantly keeping the body's priorities in order, balancing itself, and regulating itself. Despite what order we want the priorities to be in, the brain will always choose survival over comfort.

Brain Communication and Development

At birth, humans have more brain cells than at any other time in their lives. But if a neuron area in the brain doesn't work, it begins to die. In fact, this begins to happen when you are a baby. By age 5, the brain cells that didn't make connections will start to die off to ensure there is no disruption in the brain's communication. The reason most of these other neurons die off is so the precision and speed at which a child learns can be quick and efficient. The pathways that remain are constantly being activated; these pathways are called "the communication highways" in an adult.

As a child begins to grow, strong connections are made from the sensory system to the motor system. This happens when a child learns to talk and walk. There are also mirror neurons, which connect a sensory input to create the very thing it perceived. These mirror neurons fire both when a child *performs* an action, and when the child *watches* someone else perform the action. This helps children's brains develop at a rapid rate. The neuron "mirrors" the behavior of someone else, as though the child were performing the action. This is why a child often acts very similar to one or both parents—the child's neurons are mimicking the parents' actions, because the child is around them the most. Because of this, parents often have habits they hope their child will never develop, but the child does anyway. Think about this concept for a second. The possibility of talents, intelligence, personality, and mannerisms are endless, but what develops is mostly based on which parts of the brain are most often stimulated.

As people age, the brain stops functioning at the same vibrant speed it did in youth. In adulthood, the brain begins to degenerate and lose connections it once had in balance, speed, and vision; it can also start to lose memory and thought processing. This is why it is harder to learn a second language as an adult then as a child.

Brain Repair

A common belief is that the brain can heal itself. Although it's true that brain tissue can heal itself to a certain point, it is never perfectly restored to its original state. What the body does is *repair* itself. What is the difference between *healing* and *repairing*? Think of a scar. If you have a wound that has caused a lot of damage, the skin can no longer return to its normal skin tone or skin tissue texture. Instead, scar tissue is created. This new tissue may be stronger, but it is not as young and flexible as it once was. This holds true when people strain a ligament, such as one in the knee. That ligament will never be the same, but it can be repaired and function again. This also happens to the brain in many ways as you age, because the brain adapts to its repairs rather than healing and returning to perfect functioning.

What Causes Learning Disabilities

Two factors play a role in the neurological development of a child who has learning disabilities: 1) the brain receiving input from its peripheral system while out of utero, and 2) genetic coding. The parietal lobe, which manages the entire sensory system, does not develop connections until a baby is born. This is why doctors cannot know an infant's outcome until that baby grows out of the infant stage and develops brain connections. Human development is 85 percent environmental and only 15 percent genetic. Thus, no two cases are the same, as each child has a unique environment and experiences. Remember, the brain can only repair itself, not heal itself. Thus, that 85 percent environmental influence is where parents can have a greater impact on the child's long-term outcome, even when a learning disability has a genetic cause. It also means that children without genetic learning disabilities can still develop disabilities or have delays if they do not receive adequate stimulation, attention, and development as they grow.

By helping a child's sensory system provide the best input to grow and make healthy changes, a parent or caregiver helps the child's brain develop pathways and proper connections. For this reason, activities such as playing sports or learning a musical instrument are good ways to develop proper function of the brain. For example, learning to play the piano requires constant training and practice. The finger movement, the cerebellum (which coordinates everything), the temporal lobe (which is the timing sequence), and the frontal lobe (which is the actual movement command), all need to work together to make beautiful music.

PARASYMPATHETIC AND SYMPATHETIC

What are the sympathetic and parasympathetic nervous systems?

The review of homeostasis in the last chapter is the perfect lead-in to the next topic of the parasympathetic and sympathetic nervous systems.

The *sympathetic nervous system* prepares the body for emergencies and activates the fight-or-flight (or freeze) reaction of the brain when it perceives potential harm, attack, or a threat to survival. In those moments, the brain signals the adrenal glands to release a flood of hormones; blood pressure, heart rate, and blood glucose levels rise for extra energy; and there is increased blood flow to the muscles needed for fleeing or fighting. For example, this response is activated when a bear enters your camp and your body either prepares to fight the bear, quickly run away, or just freeze. Your reaction can be reflexive or linked to past experiences. In that moment, blood flow is urgently needed in the arms and legs so you can run away as quickly as possible or fight with greater strength.

Some people who suffer from insomnia or PTSD are stuck in the fight-or-flight state of hyperarousal. Anxiety and high emotions are also often the result of being caught in a sympathetic response. For example, when a panic attack strikes the heart beats rapidly and the person may have sweaty palms and a desire to get up and move or run away. These responses are also common with phobias.

The *parasympathetic nervous system* is responsible for the "rest and digest" response, which occurs when the body is at rest. This response causes the body to move blood away from the peripheral system, arms, and legs, and into the stomach. You don't want a parasympathetic response when you are running. You want this response when you are sleeping or relaxing.

Parasympathetic and sympathetic responses are regularly battling each other. One response is never 100 percent in control over the other. They are constantly balancing and checking each other, and balancing back and forth from one state to the other.

Areas of the Brain that Control Parasympathetic and Sympathetic Reponses

The area of the brain that regulates parasympathetic and sympathetic responses is in the brainstem and is part of the autonomic nervous system—a fancy word for everything that is involuntary. The brainstem consists of the midbrain, the pons, and the medulla. All input to your brain goes in and out of the brainstem.

Sympathetic response is located in the mesencephalon, or midbrain, which receives light and sound directly to its center. The reason both light and sound wake people up is because they activate the midbrain, which is the area of the brain that activates the body's flight-or-fight and awake responses. The midbrain is also where the substantia nigra is located, which produces dopamine. Dopamine is the neurotransmitter that promotes a euphoric feeling and plays a big role in reward-motivated behavior.

Sympathetic activation is steadily regulated by movement, because people need blood flow to move. Most of the midbrain's input activates two areas: 1) the frontal lobe, where deductive reasoning occurs, and 2) the basal ganglia, which is the gas and brake pedal for both voluntary and involuntary movement by the brain.

Because light, sound, movement, and reasoning all occur in, or are received by, the midbrain, people have a higher probability of activating a fight-or-flight response when they are awake. The midbrain is responsible for a sustained wakeful state, but if it increases to too high a fight-or-flight level, the person will have difficulty falling asleep. For example, when the midbrain's excitation needs to be blocked, a medically induced coma may be needed, such as with a patient in the intensive care unit due to major trauma. The coma helps the body go back into a parasympathetic state to steady the heart rate and breathing. The coma also keeps the person unconscious and not in pain, but prevents further damage through conscious movement. The midbrain is dormant while people sleep, and not responsive if a person is in a coma—either naturally or medically induced. The medulla, and parts of the pons, regulate heart rate and breathing, which can be affected by *both* sympathetic or parasympathetic responses. So, even when someone is in a coma, these areas of the brain keep the heart pumping and the lungs breathing.

The pons area of the brain also plays a role in parasympathetic and sympathetic response by serving as the message center, or planning site, but has a stronger influence on parasympathetic reactions. This area controls four cranial nerves, including the trigeminal nerve (connected to muscles of the jaw, tongue, and face sensation and pain) and the vestibular nerve (connected to balance and the head's sense of movement), which are highly connected to the medulla. The medulla regulates the heart, balance system, lungs, and vascular control with both sympathetic and parasympathetic responses. A common action that helps overall brain and the digestive function is the need to chew the food we eat. When chewing, the cranial trigeminal nerve is active, which activates the muscles of the jaw. Chewing also activates the pons, which then activates a parasympathetic response and excites the vagus nerve. The vagus nerve then sends all parasympathetic signals to the gastrointestinal tract and activates the stomach to produce the gastric enzymes and hydrochloric acid needed to break down food. This is why humans need to chew their food, and the parasympathetic response is called "rest and digest." Another aspect of the parasympathetic response involves the vestibular nucleus in the pons. The vestibular system receives input directly from the canals (for rotational movement) in each ear and two otolithic organs (for linear movement). Because of the vestibular system's connection to the parasympathetic response, it is highly connected with the vagus nerve; this is why too much rotational input (such as spinning in a circle) can make you feel nauseous.

The Role of the Eyes

Neurologists know the eyes are the window into the nervous system. This is because the eyes are the only sensory organ that activates every part of the brain. The eyes do two things. They cross (converge) and go apart (diverge), or they move in conjunction with each other. The midbrain controls eye convergence, and the pons control divergence. While asleep, the pons is hard at work. It causes the eyes to diverge, which shuts off the convergence so you can stay asleep. Yes, there is rapid alternating eye movement, but that is not involved with divergent/convergent movement.

When you wake up, the midbrain makes sure the eyes are held together. This activates a response that keeps people awake. When the eyes are crossed, or if one eye looks inward, it can cause a midbrain wind-up. This pushes a person into a constant state of fight or flight. It also decreases gut motility, creating havoc in the digestive enzymes' response and lowering blood flow to the gut. Thus, leaky gut, chronic inflammation, and a lack of food absorption often result from an eye's inability to function properly. In turn, poor food absorption results in lack of energy, which causes chronic fatigue. This example shows how different parts of the brain and body affect each other. This is important to know, because all these symptoms are the result of an overexcited sympathetic nervous system, but could be wrongly diagnosed as just a digestive problem. Remember, the gut "enteric system" is regulated by the nervous system.

The nervous system response can also be seen in the eyes with pupil response. When a person is in a parasympathetic response, the pupil decreases, or is smaller. In sympathetic response, the pupil enlarges. So, if a person is running, in a fight-or-flight state, or scared, the pupil is large. However, in some people, a large pupil occurs on one side but not on the other. When this happens, it can cause an increase in sensory input from the pupil that differs from the other. This in turn can change the brain's ability to self-regulate and balance from side to side via brain activation. If there is an imbalance to sensory input, it can also create an overactive parasympathetic or sympathetic response.

Environment also plays a big role with pupil response. For example, if a desk light is placed off to one side and a person with a pupil abnormality sits at that desk consistently enough, the light will shine more in one pupil than the other if the bridge of the nose blocks direct light from the lamp. If the desk light is on the right and a person has an abnormal pupil, the light can overstimulate the left side of the brain and create an unregulated sensory response that might increase symptoms associated with fight or flight, headaches, or fatigue.

Can a constant fight-or-flight response be stopped?

Yes. People with a chronic fight-or-flight response can be helped. Exercise is a great antidote for someone who is stuck in this state, because it activates the cerebellum. The cerebellum is located behind the brainstem, below the cortex where the spinal cord meets the brainstem. It is made up of two hemispheres. It communicates with the spinal cord, sensory system, and many other parts of the brain to oversee motor movement. It is directly connected to all three parts of the brainstem.

When you move your limbs, it fires the midbrain, which is the *sympathetic* part of the brain. However, for the body to move, your brain first has to plan and coordinate the desired movement. This planning pathway travels through the pons, and the more pons activation there is, the more *parasympathetic* responses are activated. This is why meditation allows people to relax—because the planning pathway is constantly activated with no actual movement occurring. If you move your limbs to the point of exhaustion, or to a point where you need to refuel, the parasympathetic state takes over and helps relax the sympathetic state. This is why a slow, steady walk of 30 minutes a day can help reduce the fight-or-flight state and lower anxiety levels.

All the above information shows how the sympathetic and parasympathetic are constantly balancing and checking each other. If one system is overactive for too long, it can lead to a host of gastrointestinal disturbances that can lead to fatigue and many other symptoms. Thus, achieving the proper balance between them is vital to your overall health—mentally, emotionally, and metabolically.

RECEPTOR-BASED APPROACH

What is a receptor-based approach?

Receptor based means that all sensory input activates a receptor site. It is basically a way the body codes exactly what is occurring. These receptor sites are located on an organ or body part, such as the eyes, the stomach, and the skin. Think of it this way: touch can be light or hard. This touch then gives feedback to the brain about the state of that end organ (the skin) and how the touch feels, such as either comfortable or painful. As another example, your heart is constantly sending input to your brain. The heart is the sensory organ and its receptors send signals to the brain for interpretation. If there is a breakdown to the heart's function or tissue, the brain makes adjustments to try and repair the breakdown.

As more examples, a food molecule goes into the digestive tract and is broken down until it connects to a certain receptor. So, the food is receptor specifically driven. This connection allows the enteric nervous system to break the food down further and send it through the blood stream for proper use. A signal is also sent to the central nervous system to help balance the body function. For example, once you have eaten a certain amount you feel full, which is registered in the brain via a receptor signal. This is why, depending on how well the receptor signal works, some people can eat and never feel full, or eat a tiny amount and feel full. All of these actions and responses are receptor based.

The body also has sensors. The sensors are activated by touch, movement, light, sound, smell, and or taste. Each sensor has a receptor that provides activation to the brain. These receptors have specific shapes that act as codes to fit certain molecules. Some of the senses have more than one type of receptor. For instance, light has two different types of receptors—rods (black and white) and cones (color) in the eyes. In this case, sensors are the organ itself (the eyes), but receptors are what send the signals to the brain. For example, skin is a sensor, but the variations of touch (e.g., light or heavy pressure, pain, or temperature) are the receptors that send signals to the brain.

Balance is another example of the role of sensors. Balance is maintained by the sensors in the inner ear, known as the vestibular system. These ear sensors calculate whether the body is experiencing rotational (spinning) or translational (linear) movement. This enables people to have their eyes closed and know whether they are moving forward or back, up or down, or rotating. But if the system is not balanced, you may perceive that you are moving when your eyes are open or closed, even when you are not; this can lead to chronic dizziness and even nausea.

There is nothing in the body that is not receptor based. Think of how the body regulates water and salt through your urine. If you are low in salt or high in water, your body will increase urination. If salt is high or water is low, then you will retain water and not urinate frequently. Those regulating sensors are receptors.

Sometimes the concept of receptors is hard to comprehend. When thinking about light, food, movement, and sound, one may wonder how this could all go back to receptors. Remember that there are many types of receptors. As mentioned before, the eyes have photoreceptors. Those receptors feed information to nerves and electrical stimulation through neurons. Yet the receptor itself is what activates the neurons as much as anything else. In this example, the photoreceptors are the sensory receptor that sends the image to the occipital lobe of the brain for interpretation. If the receptor is faulty, a person could have color blindness or a distortion of the image shape. Given this fact, it is possible that a person with anorexia has a visual distortion problem and not necessarily an emotional problem, or has a combination of the two; either way, anorexia is certainly a visual-perception issue. Think about when you look at distortion mirrors at an amusement park that makes you look really short and wide, or very tall and thin. Some people see the world this way. The question in these cases is, which communication channel has changed or is not functioning correctly?

The receptor system is highly complex and specific. For instance, when a sound is heard, an auditory receptor is activated, but it doesn't activate your eye receptor or photoreceptor. However, it might cause a quick chain reaction in your brain that causes your eyes to move or your heart to beat faster. Although sound, in and of itself, is not a receptor that directly activates the heart, it can indirectly activate the heart through other receptors. It is vital to understand that each receptor, or certain receptors in a sensory system, may activate certain parts of the brain, but not all parts. This can allow for specific changes to the brain by activating specific sensory pathways.

How do receptors relate to health care?

One could say that all health care providers—medical doctors, naturopaths, psychologists, dentists, chiropractors, physical therapists, massage therapists, and other health clinicians—or any professional who helps people regain their optimal health are receptor-based clinicians. The difference lies in which receptor(s) they focus on to rehabilitate a person. All of these health providers offer a viable means to get well. However, the outcome depends on:

- Which sensory receptor or nerve pathway needs to be excited for a person to no longer suffer or have pain; and

- Whether the provider can stimulate that receptor or pathway.

As examples:

- Psychologists use the limbic receptors by talking and working through difficult emotional triggers at receptors of the memory, in a safe and neutral environment.
- A chiropractor activates mechanical receptors through adjustments.
- Massage therapists activate muscle spindle receptors or Golgi tendon receptors via the muscles and fascia.
- Physical therapists perform a combination of exercises activating muscle and joint receptors.
- Surgeons may alter tissue or remove bad tissue that contains receptors that might be overactive due to the receptors' constant activation.
- Many doctors prescribe medications, which each have a specific site of activation or deactivation in the brain or gut receptors.

- Functional neurologists will use the sensory systems to alter receptor output.

Acceptance of all health professions is essential, and no methodology should be discredited. Emotional work and all other therapies have purpose. One may not work well for one person, but be perfect for someone else. Sometimes a person may simply need to ask, "Which receptor have I not tried, or what specific therapy have I not applied to my body to make it change?"

Think about all the causes of, and ways to approach, the symptoms of low back pain. It could be caused by a disc bulge, emotional stress, lack of nutrition, inflammation from a gut or bowel issue, a balance issue from a cerebellum weakness causing a muscle imbalance, a vestibular instability that regulates spinal muscle integrity, or even a lack of hearing in the ear that creates a sway to the one side due to lack of receptor input on one side. Any, or all, of these conditions could be the cause of the back pain. This is where receptor-based therapy comes into play.

What is receptor-based therapy?

The goal of receptor-based therapy is to activate the brain to create healthy homeostasis. For instance, your autonomic system decreases the amount of blood flow to the gut. Thus, if you are trying to digest food and need food for absorption, but you're in a fight-or-flight state, the digestive enzymes are not at the same level as when you are in a rest-and-digest state. In this state, no matter how much you are eating or how little you are eating, there is not enough blood to bring the food to the gastrointestinal system and on to the liver to perform its function. This leads to digestive issues. The vascular system is constantly shifting blood flow from one area to another via para vs. sympathetic changes, but blood level is fixed in the body. Therefore, the therapy needed to help this digestive issue would be to activate things that promote parasympathetic function. These could include pontine activation, such as chewing;

medulla activation, such as gargling; or deep breathing, which is a great exercise because it helps your body get into a rest-and-digest state so your body can fix its gut faster. Tying all of this together is very important in brain-based therapy. It is also important to determine what therapy is going to have the biggest impact on the brain.

Going back to the scenario of low back pain, strengthening the core muscles is a common prescription for the pain. Yet if only the abdominal muscles are activated, it may deactivate the back muscles. Will that alleviate low back pain? That would depend on the root cause of the back pain. Other possible causes could be:

- Overactive or underactive low back muscles;
- An inflammatory response from a certain cell type being activated in the stomach that causes a reflexive change in inflammation and muscle tissue; or

- An ear canal issue, because each canal has a reflex that activates certain muscles used for posture and balance. Some muscles may be turned off in the low back because of a canal being overactive, which is a reflex of the canal's activation.

How is treatment selected?

In the example of low back pain, the type of treatment needed to relieve it depends on which receptor is malfunctioning and which receptor needs to be healed, changed, or adapted for the pain to subside. This is why functional neurology is so exciting. It offers brain-based therapy with a wide variety of options for healing—not just a single option.

The key is to diagnose where the cause or breakdown is located. This is done through a full neurological exam of all the body's senses and functions, such as balance, taste, smell, sight, eye movement, coordination, walking, sound, gut sounds, heartbeat, and breathing, just to name a few. These brain rehabilitators have a whole tool bag from which to explore numerous therapies and treatment plans.

What is the best treatment plan?

Many options exist to try and help the brain work optimally. If a person doesn't have full neurological control of a reflex that might be hardwired, such as a reflex response when a hammer is tapped on the knee, then there is a problem. The automatic response should be normal muscle contraction. If the response is too fast and large, there is a problem with the central nervous system. If there is no reaction or too little muscle movement, then there is a problem with the peripheral nervous system. It is also necessary to find out whether that hardwiring is appropriate to the stimulation. In some cases, as people grow and develop, these pathways may be malformed or disconnected and become a constant problem. The problem may show up in the balance system, homeostasis of each individual cell, the gut, the brain, or even emotional stability.

There is a broad spectrum of therapies that can be used to get the brain to rehabilitate and repair itself. Some examples are sense of smell, light, colors in sequences, talking while activating a specific canal, massage, movement, gravitational pull, and touch (both light and deep). This is why massage, chiropractic adjustments, physical therapy, light therapy, psychology, medication, or surgery can all be helpful.

The main goal of receptor-based therapy is to activate a certain receptor that helps the body and mind heal from the inside out. Remember, no one therapy is bad. All doctors and therapists are doing their best to change the breakdown in a person's health by using the means they know best, but their focus must be brain based. They also need to determine whether their method of healing is the best receptor to rehabilitate the brain. If changes aren't made, then a proper referral to another type of clinician is needed to best care for the patient.

NEUROPLASTICITY

After review of the previous chapters, it is easy to see that brain rehabilitation is a complex and detailed process. It takes a lot more than merely activating a nerve cell or changing one function of the brain to repair an issue; it also takes time and practice. The term that describes this process is *neuroplasticity*, which is the brain's ability to reorganize itself by forming new neural connections throughout life. The brain is constantly adapting, but neuroplasticity takes somewhere between 3 to 5 months to make a permanent change to a programmed pathway.

How does neuroplasticity work?

Neuroplasticity was first discovered in 1950 in a study with chimpanzees. Yet it wasn't used for brain rehabilitation until 1989, and only slowly began gaining momentum in 1995. Before this, people believed the brain could not change, particularly after certain injuries, such as damage from a severe stroke or traumatic brain injury, or past a certain age.

Understanding that the brain is plastic, moldable, and changeable is a very exciting concept. Even when brain damage exists or occurs from an injury, new connections can develop and changes can be made. In fact, new connections in the brain can *always* be made. The more you work and activate a new pathway, the sooner it will become hardwired. However, neuroplasticity can be both beneficial and detrimental.

Benefits of Neuroplasticity

Neuroplasticity is beneficial because it allows functional neurologists to take a system that isn't working or hasn't been working for a long time, and in a short amount of time (3 to 5 months) alter that sensory disconnect and make new pathways. The new connection can then continue to develop and improve. Neuroplasticity also enables people to learn something new quickly, instead of taking years to learn it. For example, mathematics is a system where each concept builds upon another. So, while learning it, most children would fall behind if they missed a semester or were out of class for a month. Yet their brains can generally learn and catch up quickly, so those children can keep progressing with the rest of the class without feeling as if they are lost just because they missed one segment. Learning to throw a ball is something that can be taught very rapidly, no matter what age.

After a few trials, you don't have to think of the mechanics, your body just does them. Another example is writing in cursive. How long has it been since you wrote in cursive? For most of us, it has most likely been 5, 10, or maybe even 20 years. But if you were asked you to write the following sentence, "I love you and I'm going to heal," in cursive, you could do it because of memory recall from the neuroplasticity your brain created long ago when you learned to write in cursive.

The brain has the ability to learn, adapt, and progress. For instance, when people lose 20 lbs., all they need to do is maintain the lifestyle that helped them lose the weight and they won't regain it. If the fat comes flying back on, it's because they didn't create neuroplasticity. It isn't because they didn't have will power; neuroplasticity was simply not obtained.

Neuroplasticity is one of the greatest things about the brain, because you can damage an area but still make new connections to different areas and get the desired outcome. Neuroplasticity makes it possible for you to adapt, shift, and balance, even after serious brain trauma (e.g., a stroke, concussion, traumatic brain injury).

People are constantly changing, and neuroplasticity occurs every day of your life. Remember that the brain cannot heal itself; it repairs itself. So, if the repair is faulty, it will cause issues. The repair must be proper so it reprograms the brain to a healthy and balanced state. At that point, the change stays and you will not revert back to your old brain problems. This is why neuroplasticity is so miraculous. Again, once a change is established, you will not have your previous brain disconnect unless you experience a new trauma with an abnormal adaptation. The brain will now function in a way that produces a more desirable outcome, increased quality of life, and improved functionality with diminished suffering or pain. Although once tissue is damaged there is nothing that can regenerate it (as seen with dementia or Alzheimer's), brain functioning and quality of life *can* improve.

Drawbacks of Neuroplasticity

Neuroplasticity can also be detrimental when it creates new pathways that cause problems. Consider, for instance, the impact of staring at a smart phone, TV, computer, or video game for hours each day. This can create a midbrain wind-up or increased dopamine levels, which is part of the addiction pathway. That is why video gaming can become addictive or tantrums can occur when a child is asked to stop playing. The light from long, sustained screen time also activates the body's photoreceptors, which then alters the way the pupil reacts to light; this can lead to headaches or migraines. The prolonged screen light can also cause a heightened sensitivity to light when it travels into the upper part of the midbrain. This is why it's common for headache sufferers to stay in a dark room, and people with a concussion want to turn off all electronics and decrease sound. Therefore, if a person has consistently been exposed to visual electronics, he or she will have a wound-up midbrain that is very plastic. Then if a head trauma occurs, which damages the brainstem, that person's plastic, overactive midbrain becomes an even bigger problem!

Things to Watch for

Because most people in today's world can't (or won't) completely give up smart phones, computers, televisions, or video games, there are ways to rehabilitate different parts of the brain to put symptoms in check without removing the stimulation (i.e., screen time).

It is also important not only to activate the brain, but to remove stimulation that is bad or normally on one side. However, the goal of this type of rehabilitation is not to become ambidextrous, as right or left handedness is important to the brain's development. Right-handed people use more of the left motor strip of the frontal lobe and vice versa for left-handed people. Remember that people are affected by both genetics and pre-programmed systems, such as handedness, and these systems must be used to develop proper function. So please, don't change your handedness in hopes of becoming more right (creative) or left (analytical) brain dominant. There are other ways to improve creativity and become more logical.

In today's world, there is much debate about whether cell phones and laptops are affecting our genes or overall health. From a functional neurology standpoint, having a computer on your lap causes you to look down and/or bend your head down, which can cause an increase of midbrain activity; this in turn activates greater sympathetic nervous system output. Keeping your head in that position also puts more stress on the neck muscles if maintained for too long, which gives feedback to your brain from the neck extensors (the muscles on the back of your neck). The difference in muscle activation and stimulation may alter balance, which can cause a host of issues. As for cell phones, the questions are which pocket do you carry it in, and is it on vibrate? The constant input from the phone may be altering your balance of sensory input from left to right. People sometimes feel the ring of a phone call or vibration in their pocket from a call or text that didn't actually occur. That is caused by overactive sensory input, meaning you sense something that didn't happen.

Because cell phones are a way of life, here are some tips for keeping your sensory input balanced while using one:

- Avoid sitting or lying down while on your phone.
- Walk around while you talk.
- Put it on speaker phone whenever possible.
- Use headphones so sound comes in equally to both ears.
- Change up the hand you use to hold your phone and the ear to which you hold it.
- Move your feet while talking.
- Draw a figure eight with your free arm while on your phone.
- Move your feet in a cross-crawl tap.

These are all things that can change how your brain adapts to the constant input from your cell phone, keeping you balanced and functioning better. The same tips apply to constant use of computers, video games, and television watching—keep your body moving, change positions after sitting for a while, and take breaks.

How long does brain rehabilitation take?

Neuroplasticity and brain rehabilitation take time and patience. Think about how long it takes to learn a new skill, such as playing an instrument, learning a second language, or becoming good at a sport. Another example is how long it takes the body to get in shape, build muscles, or lose weight. It simply takes a great deal of time, dedication, and commitment to achieve lasting changes. The brain requires the same level of commitment to create long-term changes. Remember, everything you want to learn or do is controlled by your brain. As one example, if people with diabetes change their diet and exercise to reduce symptoms, it will take the brain time to change how the blood sugars and pancreas react, how the body digests food, the body's reaction time, and how long the muscles take to uptake glucose for energy and utilize fuel.

Muscle development is what everyone seeks to establish in an exercise program, and functional neurologists, or brain-based therapists, do the same thing with the brain. They use very targeted exercises to help the brain build strength and stability for its new pathways and connections. These exercises are done several times daily for 3 to 5 months to achieve a lasting change to that function, though it may be great or small. The progression will not only improve a single outcome but can improve multiple outcomes; these improvements can be seen well after the 5 months.

The Constantly Changing Brain

The miraculous thing about the brain is that it is *constantly* changing. The brain can always learn new concepts and develop new skills. Even someone who is 95 years old can learn a new language. The brain can also always make new connections. Patients who have brain damage, due to a tumor or an accident, may have areas of the brain that no longer work. However, there are "highways" in the brain that connect one part to another. This means that with the right targeted exercises, one part of the brain can be rerouted to connect to another part, and then another. Rerouting the connections can create a new pathway that bypasses the damaged area. The end result is a new connection that the brain wouldn't have manifested on its own, simply because it was used to doing things the old way.

Giving the brain new input and stimulation, in the right order, can help it to once again function normally. Remember, this takes time—sometimes months and even a year, because neuroplasticity builds upon neuroplasticity. Once you change the brain, new connections are being made to those newly developed pathways. It is not easy to change a pathway that has been hardwired in a certain way for many years, *but it is possible*. Therefore, patience and commitment are a necessary part of rehabbing the brain.

What helps create neuroplasticity and brain changes?

Daily exercise, eating healthy foods, and eliminating substances that cause inflammation (such as artificial sweeteners, processed foods, and genetically modified foods) are also essential aspects of neuroplasticity. Given the average life span of humans, the brain needs to last a long time. So, the better you hardwire it and the more you take care of it—not just occasionally, but consistently day after day—the better, and longer, it will work for you.

Finding the area (or areas) of the brain that isn't connecting is the key to regaining good health. Here are two examples:

- Children with learning disabilities require evaluations of which areas of the brain are not connecting, or whether there are portions that are not developing. Questions that functional neurologists consider include: Is there a stimulant that is over-activating part of the brain, or is stimulation needed to activate a weak area of the brain? Are there areas of the brain that have not been activated at all?

- With anxiety, gut function must be evaluated, including diet or the lack of nutritional support. Questions to consider include: Is the person stuck in a fight-or-flight stage neurologically, and what might be the causes of that disconnect? Is there an emotional trigger, such as a post-traumatic stress disorder? What is in their environment that they can't get away from? Is it a lack of sleep? Is it a hormonal imbalance? And, how do all these issues tie together?

The answers to these questions may be the missing links to creating neuroplasticity and changing the brain's usual dysfunction— both voluntary and involuntarily. Remember that the brain's hierarchy is consistently being chosen to keep you alive. Thus, the goal of brain rehabilitation is to establish homeostasis so that all things work together as one healthy whole.

An easy way to understand neuroplasticity is to look at how the leg moves. A person who fidgets and constantly taps the foot every day—over, and over, and over again—will eventually program the brain so it keeps tapping automatically—such as a nervous habit or tic. Neuroplasticity is also easy to see in athletes and musicians, where specific movements they practice each day become automatic. This creation of automatic movement is termed *muscle memory*. But is it really a muscle memory, or is it a connection memory? Most likely it is the brain's circuitry or programming that has the memory. Memories are stored in the brain, and individual muscles have receptor sites. Therefore, muscle memory doesn't truly exist. It is actually cerebellum autopilot, or your brain doing what you have programmed it to do.

For example, an athlete who is first learning and training uses a great deal of cerebellum activity. But after practicing specific moves for hours each day, those moves become a reaction or a reflex. The muscles no longer require much cerebellum activity to perform those practiced moves. Instead, those skills become auto-pilot receptor reflexes. This is also true with musicians. The cerebellum works much harder and is highly activated when a musician is learning a new song. Then the cerebellum hardly works at all when a performer is playing a memorized song, and can instead focus on another aspect of performing, such as singing and entertaining.

The Future

Science and medicine have only begun to scratch the surface of neuroplasticity. There is so much more to explore. Ten, 20, or even 30 years from now, there will be a wealth of understanding about how the brain can change, be reprogrammed, and become more efficient. Health will be obtained from the top down and inside out, and brain rehabilitation will become tremendously advanced and advantageous to chronic illnesses.

CONCLUSION

Given the possibilities that neuroplasticity make possible, the goal of every practitioner—especially functional neurologists—is to give the right therapy, in the right sequence, at the right time. Once the right formula is established, this prescribed therapy needs to be a patient's priority for complete brain rehabilitation to occur. It takes work and commitment on the part of the patient. Doing the prescribed brain exercises can be time consuming and difficult, but the end result is a brain that is forever changed.

The intent of this booklet is to educate patients about what it takes to rehabilitate the brain. You have learned that the brain is receptor based. You also now understand that all communication between the immune, enteric nervous, limbic-emotional, and endocrine systems is regulated and balanced by the central nervous system. The central nervous system is highly connected and receives input through receptors from the sensory systems, both internal and external. You hopefully also realize that your sensory system has an impact on how your brain functions and regulates itself.

Poor health is rarely caused by a genetic component. Most illness is caused by an environmental factor. For example, many behavioral problems and certain illnesses in children are less genetic and more environmental. Also, environmental factors can come into play and change health conditions that have run in a family line for generations. For example, dementia or diabetes may run in a family, but environment plays a bigger role in how and whether these illnesses develop than does the family's gene pool. Even if a person is genetically predisposed to diabetes, it can be kept at bay through many environmental factors, such as exercise, diet, and medication. Also, recent studies show that most cases of Alzheimer's disease have environmental causes.

The only way to know whether a health condition can be altered is to activate new brain connections or change the environment, and then see whether the symptoms change. Without going into great detail, the central nervous system regulates everything, even whether genes are expressed or not expressed.

Many new studies show that discrepancies on one side of the brain or the other can lead to dysfunction. There are many functions of our lives that are controlled by only one side of the brain. For example, the language center is in the left hemisphere. Thus, if a person has a stroke in the left side, they typically can't communicate verbally. But if the stroke is on the right, the person can still communicate. Other examples are that the immune system can be stimulated by left-brain activity, and stimulation of the right side of the brain can dampen it.

All sensory input will first excite the brain's programed designated area. Then the nerve impulse will either excite another area to promote more action, and/or stimulate another impulse that will diminish or stop the action. This imbalance of the left and right brain is commonly observed when treating patients with learning disabilities, movement disorders (tremors), behavior problems, and chronic pain.

How to Create Lasting Brain Changes

Finding the correct receptor is fundamental to creating change. As one example, when someone has an autoimmune disease, the clinician must ask what can be done to change or stop the body from attacking itself. Is it genetic, and can it be changed?

In this case, the clinician must: 1) locate the parts of the brain that aren't working, 2) reconnect those parts, and 3) get them working the right way. Some common ways to speed brain rehabilitation for an autoimmune disease include:

- Increased activation of the right brain that can dampen the immune system's response.
- Medications that help lesson immune responses.
- Eliminating inflammatory foods from one's diet.
- Exercise to help decrease inflammation and increase oxygen exchange.
- Proper sleep to regulate cortisol levels and blood sugars.
- Supplements for any deficiencies that the body might have, such as with anemias.
- And, the list goes on, and on, and on.

A host of things are evaluated before rehabbing the brain, such as balance, eye movement, cranial nerve testing, blood labs, and sensory evaluations. This is because the most important thing is to properly diagnose and get the correct combination of stimulation that inspires repair. The right therapy, at the right time, and in the correct sequence, can generate the highest level of recovery possible.

Summary

Functional neurologists expect a certain outcome from brain rehabilitation because of neuroplasticity. The brain can be molded and changed to meet the desired outcomes, because the brain adapts accordingly to new stimulation. Once a patient starts doing the assigned exercises, there is always an adaptation phase, which takes time. The end objective is to rehabilitate the brain and get it functioning at its fullest potential.

As a functional neurologist, the work of brain rehabilitation is an absolute pleasure. Watching progress unfold and the positive changes that occur in a patient's life is an unparalleled experience. As you embark on your journey to brain change, don't give up.

Keep trying new things and your healing will occur.

RESOURCES ABOUT NUTRITION AND THE BRAIN

Kharrazian, D. (2013). *Why Isn't My Brain Working?: A Revolutionary Understanding of Brain Decline and Effective Strategies to Recover Your Brain's Health.* Dallas, TX: Elephant Press.

Perlmutter, D. & Loberg, K. (2015). *Brain Maker: The Power of Gut Microbes to Heal and Protect Your Brain–for Life.* Boston, MA: Little, Brown and Company.

Perlmutter, D. & Loberg, K. (2013). *Grain Brain: The Surprising Truth about Wheat, Carbs, and Sugar--Your Brain's Silent Killers.* Boston, MA: Little, Brown and Company.

Mitchell, W. (2015). *The Unbreakable Brain: Shield Your Brain From Cognitive Decline...For Life!* Austin, TX: Merritt Wellness Center.

51020747R00055

Made in the USA
San Bernardino, CA
10 July 2017